KETO AIR FRYE

Toasted Nuts edition

LINDSAY ROW

Contents

Toasted Walnuts	50
Pepper Roasted Walnuts	52
Candied Walnuts	54
Roasted Walnuts	56
Cinnamon Roasted Walnuts	58
Rosemary Toasted Walnuts	60
Maple Roasted Walnuts	62
Espresso Roasted Walnuts	64
Rosemary Macadamias	66
Spiced Macadamia Nuts	68
Chile Macadamia Nuts	71
Maple Macadamia Nuts	73
Rosemary Brazil Nuts	75
Brazil Nuts Mix	78
Espresso Roasted Cashews	81
Chile Brazilian Nuts	83
Garlic Macadamia Nuts	85
Chai Spiced Nuts	87
Gingerbread Glazed Nuts	90
Sesame Cashew Clusters	92
Chilli Lime Cashews	94
Chocolate Pecans	97
Chocolate Dipped Walnuts	99

SMOKEY ROASTED PISTACHIOS

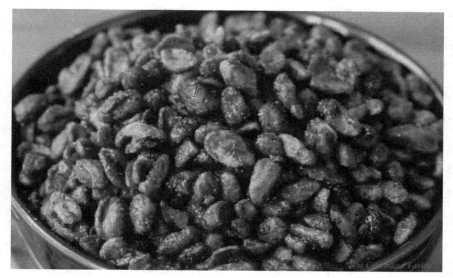

Serves: 6-8

Prep Time: 14 mins

Cook Time: 15 mins

Ingredients:

- 2 teaspoons olive oil
- 2 teaspoons butter melted
- 1 tablespoon choc zero maple syrup
- 1 tablespoon brown swerve
- 1 teaspoon applewood smoked salt

- ½ teaspoon cinnamon
- 8 oz. shelled unsalted pistachios

Directions:

1. Mix olive oil, butter, maple syrup, swerve, salt, cinnamon, and smoked salt in a bowl.
2. Toss in pistachios and mix well to coat.
3. At 300 degrees F, preheat your Air Fryer.
4. Grease the Air Fryer basket with vegetable oil.
5. Spread the nuts in the Air Fryer basket and spray them with cooking oil.
6. Air fry these nuts for 15 minutes and toss once cooked halfway through. Serve.

Nutritional Values:

Calories: 181, Fat: 16.3g, Carb: 7g, Protein: 6g

MAPLE ROASTED PISTACHIOS

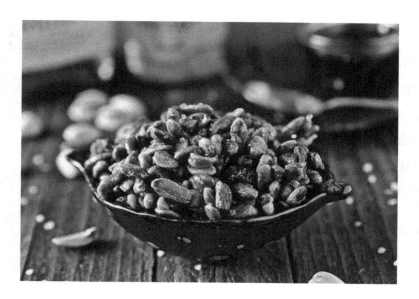

Serves: 6-8

Prep Time: 14 mins

Cook Time: 15 mins

Ingredients:

- 1 cup pistachios
- 1 teaspoon grapeseed oil
- 1/2 tablespoons choc zero maple syrup

- Salt

Directions:

1. Toss pistachios with oil, salt and maple syrup in a bowl.
2. At 300 degrees F, preheat your Air Fryer.
3. Grease the Air Fryer basket with vegetable oil.
4. Spread the nuts in the Air Fryer basket and spray them with cooking oil.
5. Air fry these nuts for 15 minutes and toss once cooked halfway through. Serve.

Nutritional Values:

Calories: 140, Fat: 16.3g, Carb: 7.7g, Protein: 18g

BERBERE ROASTED PISTACHIOS

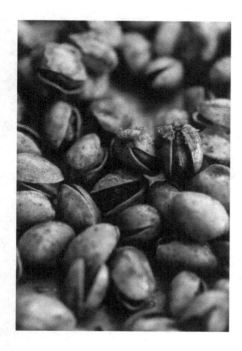

Serves: 6

8 Prep Time: 14 mins

Cook Time: 20 mins

Ingredients:

- 1 tablespoon choc zero maple syrup

- 1 tablespoon pistachio oil
- 1 tablespoon lemon juice
- 1 tablespoon frontier berbere blend
- 1/2 teaspoon salt
- Zest from 1 lemon
- 2 cups raw pistachios in the shell

Directions:

1. Mix maple syrup, pistachio oil, lemon juice, berbere blend, salt, and lemon zest
2. Toss in pistachios and mix well to coat.
3. At 300 degrees F, preheat your Air Fryer.
4. Grease the Air Fryer basket with vegetable oil.
5. Spread the nuts in the Air Fryer basket and spray them with cooking oil.
6. Air fry these nuts for 20 minutes and toss once cooked halfway through. Serve.

Nutritional Values:

Calories: 144, Fat: 20.2g, Carb: 6.9g, Protein: 9g

LEMON SAFFRON ROASTED PISTACHIOS

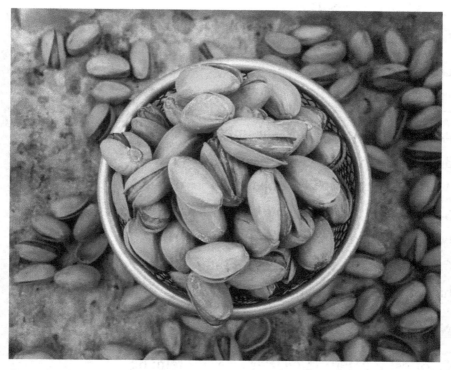

Serves: 6-8

Prep Time: 14 mins

Cook Time: 25 mins

Ingredients:

- 3 cups raw pistachios (in the shell)
- juice of 3 lemons
- 3 teaspoons salt
- 1 pinch saffron

Directions:

1. Mix saffron with salt and lemon juice in mortar with pestle.
2. Toss pistachios with this mixture in a bowl.
3. At 325 degrees F, preheat your Air Fryer.
4. Grease the Air Fryer basket with vegetable oil.
5. Spread the nuts in the Air Fryer basket and spray them with cooking oil.
6. Air fry these nuts for 25 minutes and toss once cooked halfway through. Serve.

Nutritional Values:

Calories: 132, Fat: 14.9g, Carb: 7g, Protein: 6g

ZAATAR PEANUTS

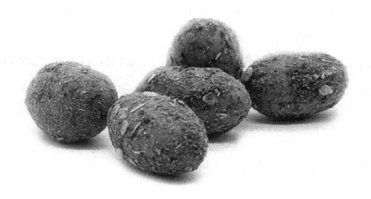

Serves: 6-8

Prep Time: 14 mins

Cook Time: 25 mins

Ingredients:

- 2 cups peanuts

- 2 teaspoons olive oil
- 2 teaspoons Za'atar seasoning

Directions:

1. Mix peanuts with zaatar with olive oil in a bowl.
2. At 300 degrees F, preheat your Air Fryer.
3. Grease the Air Fryer basket with vegetable oil.
4. Spread the nuts in the Air Fryer basket and spray them with cooking oil.
5. Air fry these nuts for 25 minutes and toss once cooked halfway through. Serve.

Nutritional Values:

Calories: 242, Fat: 16.3g, Carb: 9g, Protein: 6g

TOASTED CECCHI AND PISTACHIOS

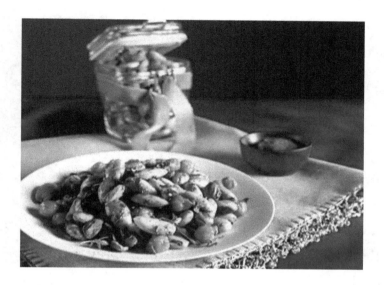

Serves: 6-8

Prep Time: 14 mins

Cook Time: 30 mins

Ingredients:

- 1 tablespoon olive oil, plus 3 tablespoons
- 1 ½ cup shelled pistachios
- 1 ½ cup raw almonds
- 1 tablespoon swerve

- 1 tablespoon chopped fresh rosemary leaves
- 1 tablespoon chopped fresh thyme leaves
- 1 teaspoon coarse salt
- 1/2 teaspoon cayenne

Directions:

1. Mix olive oil, swerve, rosemary, thyme, salt and cayenne in a bowl.
2. Toss in pistachios and mix well to coat.
3. At 400 degrees F, preheat your Air Fryer.
4. Grease the Air Fryer basket with vegetable oil.
5. Spread the nuts in the Air Fryer basket and spray them with cooking oil.
6. Air fry these nuts for 30 minutes and toss once cooked halfway through. Serve.

Nutritional Values:

Calories: 395, Fat: 17.1g, Carb: 8.1g, Protein: 10g

PAPRIKA LIME PISTACHIOS

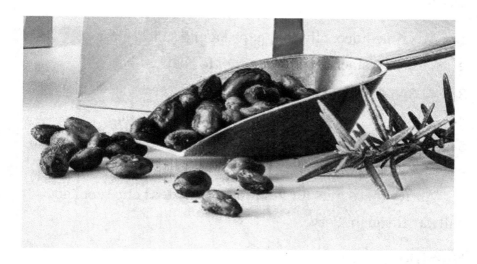

Serves: 6-8

Prep Time: 14 mins

Cook Time: 22 mins

Ingredients:

- ¼ cup fresh lime juice
- 2 tablespoons olive oil
- 2 teaspoons hot paprika
- 2 teaspoons salt

- 3 cups (1 lb.) Raw shelled pistachios

Directions:

1. Mix lime juice, olive oil, paprika and salt in a bowl.
2. Toss in pistachios and mix well to coat.
3. At 325 degrees F, preheat your Air Fryer.
4. Grease the Air Fryer basket with vegetable oil.
5. Spread the nuts in the Air Fryer basket and spray them with cooking oil.
6. Air fry these nuts for 22 minutes and toss once cooked halfway through. Serve.

Nutritional Values:

Calories: 144, Fat: 20g, Carb: 7g, Protein: 9g

CINNAMON PISTACHIOS

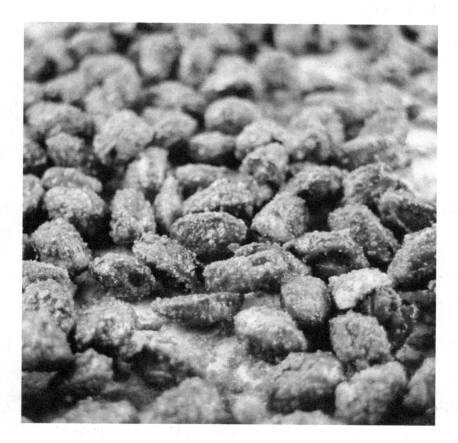

Serves: 6-8

Prep Time: 14 mins

Cook Time: 25 mins

Ingredients:

- 1 egg white
- 1 teaspoon vanilla
- 3 cups pistachios
- 1/2 cup white swerve
- 1/2 cup brown swerve
- 1/4 teaspoon salt
- 1 teaspoon McCormick ground cinnamon

Directions:

1. Mix egg white, vanilla, swerve, salt, and cinnamon in a bowl.
2. Toss in pistachios and mix well to coat.
3. At 350 degrees F, preheat your Air Fryer.
4. Grease the Air Fryer basket with vegetable oil.
5. Spread the nuts in the Air Fryer basket and spray them with cooking oil.
6. Air fry these nuts for 25 minutes and toss once cooked halfway through. Serve.

Nutritional Values:

Calories: 134, Fat: 18g, Carb: 4.8g, Protein: 18g

CINNAMON HAZELNUTS

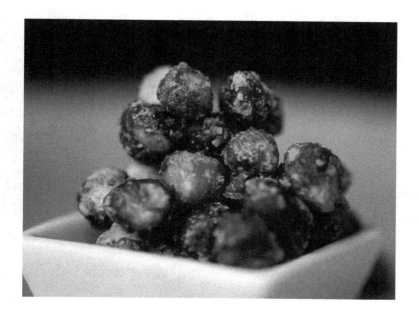

Serves: 6-8

Prep Time: 14 mins

Cook Time: 25 mins

Ingredients:

- 1 egg white
- 1 tablespoon water

- 2 1/4 cups hazelnut
- 1/2 cup white swerve
- 1/4 teaspoon salt
- 1 1/2 teaspoons ground cinnamon

Directions:

1. Beat egg white with water, swerve, salt and cinnamon in a bowl.
2. Toss in hazelnuts and mix well to coat.
3. At 350 degrees F, preheat your Air Fryer.
4. Grease the Air Fryer basket with vegetable oil.
5. Spread the nuts in the Air Fryer basket and spray them with cooking oil.
6. Air fry these nuts for 25 minutes and toss once cooked halfway through. Serve.

Nutritional Values:

Calories: 194, Fat: 13.8g, Carb: 5.7g, Protein: 6g

SALT-ROASTED PECANS

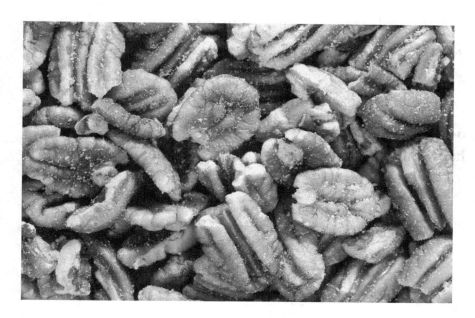

Serves: 6-8

Prep Time: 14 mins

Cook Time: 15 mins

Ingredients:

- 2 cups pecan halves
- 3 tablespoons unsalted butter, melted
- 1 1/4 teaspoons Salt, to taste

Directions:

1. Mix pecans with salt, and butter in a bowl.
2. At 325 degrees F, preheat your Air Fryer.
3. Grease the Air Fryer basket with vegetable oil.
4. Spread the nuts in the Air Fryer basket and spray them with cooking oil.
5. Air fry these nuts for 15 minutes and toss once cooked halfway through. Serve.

Nutritional Values:

Calories: 132, Fat: 16.3g, Carb: 5.9g, Protein: 6g

MAPLE ROASTED PECANS

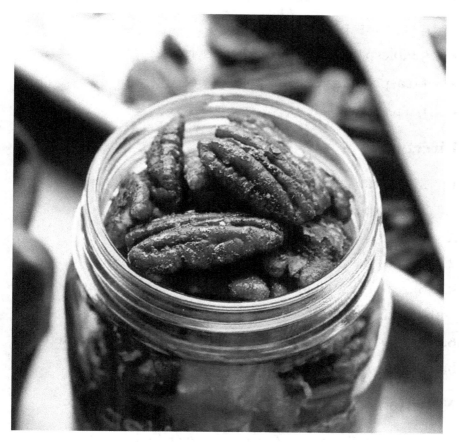

Serves: 6-8

Prep Time: 14 mins

Cook Time: 10 mins

Ingredients:

- 4 cups raw pecans
- 3 tablespoons choc zero maple syrup
- 1 teaspoon ground cinnamon
- 1/2 teaspoon salt

Directions:

1. Mix pecans, maple syrup, cinnamon and salt in a bowl.
2. Toss in pecans and mix well to coat.
3. At 400 degrees F, preheat your Air Fryer.
4. Grease the Air Fryer basket with vegetable oil.
5. Spread the nuts in the Air Fryer basket and spray them with cooking oil.
6. Air fry these nuts for 10 minutes and toss once cooked halfway through. Serve.

Nutritional Values:

Calories: 157, Fat: 16.3g, Carb: 7.9g, Protein: 6g

BUTTER ROASTED PECANS

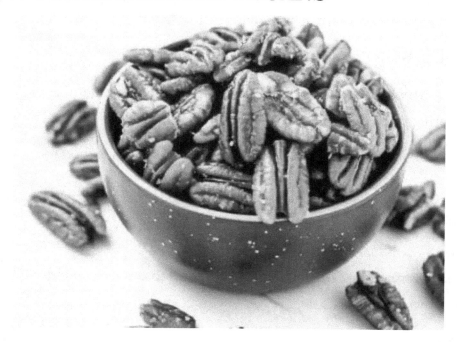

Serves: 6-8

Prep Time: 14 mins

Cook Time: 12 mins

Ingredients:

- 5 cups of pecan halves
- 1/4 cup butter
- 1 1/2 teaspoons salt

- 1 tablespoon choc zero maple syrup
- 1 tablespoon fresh sage, chopped

Directions:

1. Mix butter, salt, and maple syrup in a saucepan and cook until golden brown.
2. Stir in sage and pecans then mix well.
3. At 350 degrees F, preheat your Air Fryer.
4. Grease the Air Fryer basket with vegetable oil.
5. Spread the nuts in the Air Fryer basket and spray them with cooking oil.
6. Air fry these nuts for 12 minutes and toss once cooked halfway through. Serve.

Nutritional Values:

Calories: 283, Fat: 20.2g, Carb: 4.8g, Protein: 10g

BERBERE MACADAMIA NUTS

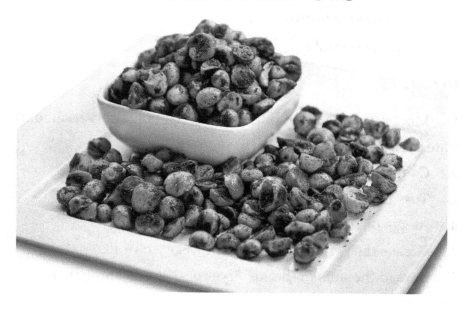

Serves: 6-8

Prep Time: 14 mins

Cook Time: 15 mins

Ingredients:

- 2 cups MACADAMIA NUTS
- 1 1/2 tablespoons unsalted butter
- 2 teaspoons ras el hanout
- Large pinch cayenne pepper

- 1 1/4 teaspoons salt
- 3 tablespoons brown swerve
- 1 tablespoon water

Directions:

1. Mix butter, ras el hanout, cayenne pepper, swerve, salt and water in a saucepan.
2. Cook this mixture to a boil and allow it to cool.
3. Toss in macadamia nuts and mix well to coat.
4. At 375 degrees F, preheat your Air Fryer.
5. Grease the Air Fryer basket with vegetable oil.
6. Spread the nuts in the Air Fryer basket and spray them with cooking oil.
7. Air fry these nuts for 15 minutes and toss once cooked halfway through. Serve.

Nutritional Values:

Calories: 140, Fat: 16g, Carb: 8.3 g, Protein: 18g

ESPRESSO ROASTED CASHEWS

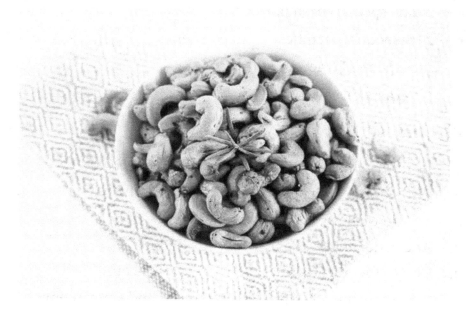

Serves: 6-8

Prep Time: 14 mins

Cook Time: 45 mins

Ingredients:

- 4 cups cashews
- 2 egg whites
- 1 teaspoon vanilla

- 3/4 cup brown swerve
- 2 tablespoons cocoa powder
- 2 teaspoons instant espresso powder
- 1 teaspoon of dried chipotle pepper
- 1/2 teaspoon salt

Directions:

1. Beat egg whites with vanilla, swerve, cocoa powder, espresso powder, chipotle pepper and salt in a bowl.
2. Toss in cashews and mix well to coat.
3. At 275 degrees F, preheat your Air Fryer.
4. Grease the Air Fryer basket with vegetable oil.
5. Spread the nuts in the Air Fryer basket and spray them with cooking oil.
6. Air fry these nuts for 45 minutes and toss once cooked halfway through. Serve.

Nutritional Values:

Calories: 134, Fat: 17.4g, Carb: 8.1g, Protein: 9g

MOROCCAN PECANS

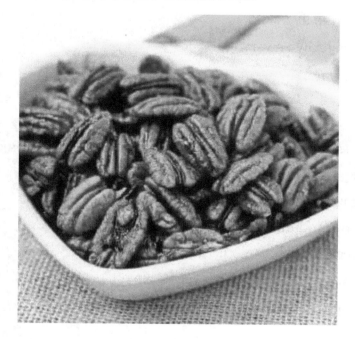

Serves: 6-8

Prep Time: 14 mins

Cook Time: 15 mins

Ingredients:

- 2 cups pecans
- 1 1/2 tablespoons unsalted butter
- 2 teaspoons ras el hanout

- Large pinch cayenne pepper
- 1 1/4 teaspoons salt
- 3 tablespoons brown swerve
- 1 tablespoon water

Directions:

1. Mix butter, ras el hanout, cayenne pepper, swerve, salt and water in a saucepan.
2. Cook this mixture to a boil and allow it to cool.
3. Toss in pecans and mix well to coat.
4. At 375 degrees F, preheat your Air Fryer.
5. Grease the Air Fryer basket with vegetable oil.
6. Spread the nuts in the Air Fryer basket and spray them with cooking oil.
7. Air fry these nuts for 15 minutes and toss once cooked halfway through. Serve.

Nutritional Values:

Calories: 242, Fat: 20g, Carb: 7.7g, Protein: 6g

TOASTED ROSEMARY PECANS

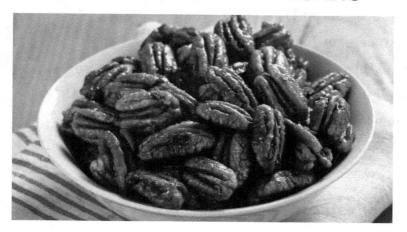

Serves: 6-8

Prep Time: 14 mins

Cook Time: 15 mins

Ingredients:

- 4 cups pecan halves
- 4 tablespoons unsalted butter
- 1 ½ teaspoons salt
- 1 teaspoon dried rosemary
- ½ teaspoon swerve

Directions:

1. Mix butter, salt, swerve and rosemary in a bowl.

2. Toss in pecans and mix well to coat.

3. At 250 degrees F, preheat your Air Fryer.

4. Grease the Air Fryer basket with vegetable oil.

5. Spread the nuts in the Air Fryer basket and spray them with cooking oil.

6. Air fry these nuts for 15 minutes and toss once cooked halfway through. Serve.

Nutritional Values:

Calories: 194, Fat: 16.3g, Carb: 7g, Protein: 6g

SPICY SESAME WALNUTS

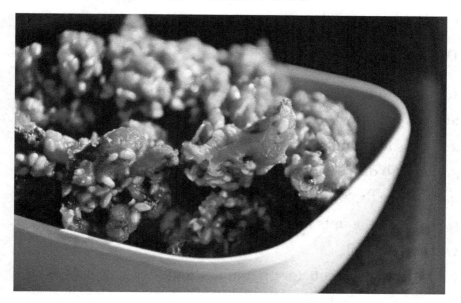

Serves: 6-8

Prep Time: 14 mins

Cook Time: 20 mins

Ingredients:

- 1-pound walnut halves
- 1 cup swerve
- ½ cup water
- ⅔ cup sesame seeds

- 1 ¼ teaspoons cayenne pepper
- ½ teaspoon salt

Directions:

1. Mix walnut, swerve, water, sesame seeds, cayenne pepper, and salt in a bowl.
2. Toss in walnuts and mix well to coat.
3. At 350 degrees F, preheat your Air Fryer.
4. Grease the Air Fryer basket with vegetable oil.
5. Spread the nuts in the Air Fryer basket and spray them with cooking oil.
6. Air fry these nuts for 20 minutes and toss once cooked halfway through. Serve.

Nutritional Values:

Calories: 157, Fat: 14.9g, Carb: 6.9g, Protein: 10g

SAVORY SESAME PECANS

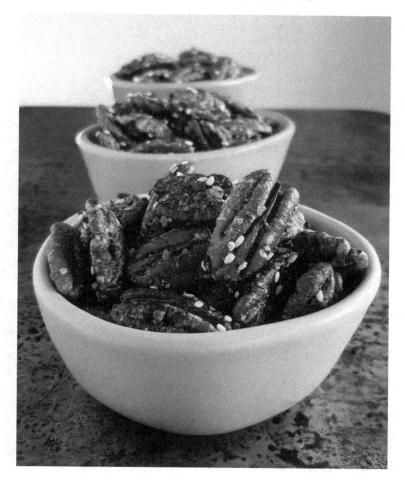

Serves: 6-8

Prep Time: 14 mins

Cook Time: 25 mins

Ingredients:

- 1 lb. pecans raw
- 4 tablespoons butter melted
- ⅔ cup sesame seeds
- 2 tablespoons pure choc zero maple syrup
- 1 ½ teaspoons chili powder
- 1 teaspoon paprika
- ¼ - ½ teaspoons cayenne pepper
- ½ teaspoons garlic powder
- 1 ¼ teaspoons salt to taste
- ¼ teaspoons cinnamon

Directions:

1. Mix butter with maple syrup, chili powder, paprika, cayenne pepper, sesame seeds, garlic powder, salt and cinnamon in a bowl.
2. Toss in walnuts and mix well to coat.
3. At 300 degrees F, preheat your Air Fryer.
4. Grease the Air Fryer basket with vegetable oil.

5.   Spread the nuts in the Air Fryer basket and spray them with cooking oil.

6.   Air fry these nuts for 25 minutes and toss once cooked halfway through. Serve.

Nutritional Values:

Calories: 132, Fat: 16.3g, Carb: 4.8g, Protein: 18g

CINNAMON WALNUTS

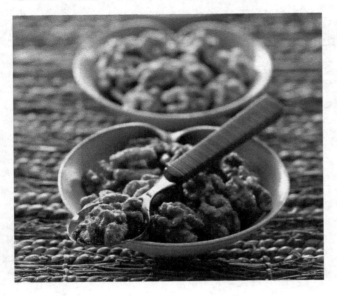

Serves: 6-8

Prep Time: 14 mins

Cook Time: 20 mins

Ingredients:

- 1 cup raw walnut halves
- 1 teaspoon ground cinnamon
- 3 tablespoons choc zero maple syrup
- Pinch of salt

Directions:

1. Mix maple syrup, salt and cinnamon in a suitable bowl.
2. Toss in walnuts and mix well to coat.
3. At 350 degrees F, preheat your Air Fryer.
4. Grease the Air Fryer basket with vegetable oil.
5. Spread the nuts in the Air Fryer basket and spray them with cooking oil.
6. Air fry these nuts for 20 minutes and toss once cooked halfway through. Serve.

Nutritional Values:

Calories: 144, Fat: 18.6g, Carb: 5.9g, Protein: 6g

SWEET SESAME WALNUTS

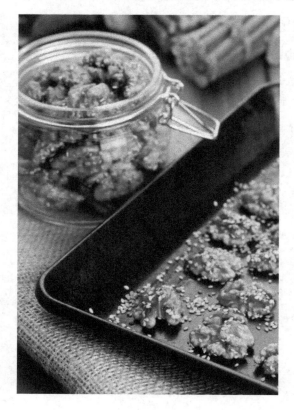

Serves: 6-8

Prep Time: 14 mins

Cook Time: 10 mins

Ingredients:

- 1 cup untoasted walnut halves
- 1/4 teaspoon salt
- 1/4 teaspoon cumin
- 1/4 teaspoon cayenne pepper
- 1/4 teaspoon white pepper powder
- 1/4 cup swerve
- 1 tablespoon water
- ½ tablespoon butter
- 2 tablespoons sesame seeds

Directions:

1. Mix salt, cumin, cayenne pepper, white pepper powder, swerve, water, and butter in a bowl.
2. Toss in walnuts and mix well to coat.
3. At 300 degrees F, preheat your Air Fryer.
4. Grease the Air Fryer basket with vegetable oil.
5. Spread the nuts in the Air Fryer basket and spray them with cooking oil.
6. Air fry these nuts for 10 minutes and toss once cooked halfway through.
7. Drizzle sesame seeds on top of the nuts. Serve.

Nutritional Values:

Calories: 134, Fat: 18g, Carb: 6.2g, Protein: 9g

MOROCCAN SPICED WALNUTS

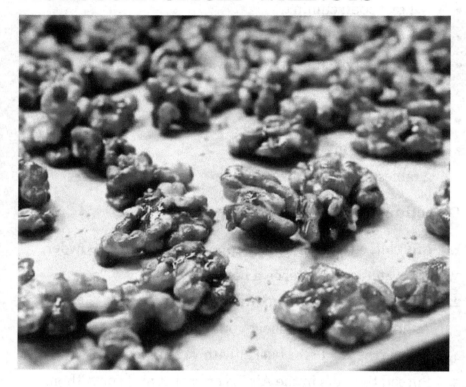

Serves: 6-8

Prep Time: 14 mins

Cook Time: 15 mins

Ingredients:

- 2 cups walnuts
- 1 1/2 tablespoons unsalted butter
- 2 teaspoons ras el hanout
- Large pinch cayenne pepper
- 1 1/4 teaspoons salt
- 3 tablespoons brown swerve
- 1 tablespoon water

Directions:

1. Mix butter, ras el hanout, cayenne pepper, swerve, salt and water in a saucepan.
2. Cook this mixture to a boil and allow it to cool.
3. Toss in walnuts and mix well to coat.
4. At 375 degrees F, preheat your Air Fryer.
5. Grease the Air Fryer basket with vegetable oil.
6. Spread the nuts in the Air Fryer basket and spray them with cooking oil.
7. Air fry these nuts for 15 minutes and toss once cooked halfway through.
8. Serve.

Nutritional Values:

Calories: 281, Fat: 17.1g, Carb: 9g, Protein: 6g

SPICED ROASTED WALNUTS

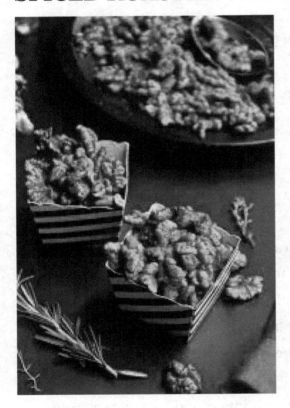

Serves: 6-8

Prep Time: 14 mins

Cook Time: 10 mins

Ingredients:

- 3 cups walnut halves
- 2 tablespoons olive oil
- 1/4 teaspoon ground coriander
- 1/2 teaspoon ground cumin
- 1 1/2 teaspoons smoked paprika
- 1/2 teaspoon red chili flakes
- 1 tablespoon fresh thyme, minced
- 1 teaspoon fresh rosemary, minced

Directions:

1. Mix olive oil, coriander, cumin, paprika, chili flakes, thyme, and rosemary in a bowl.
2. Toss in walnuts and mix well to coat.
3. At 350 degrees F, preheat your Air Fryer.
4. Grease the Air Fryer basket with vegetable oil.
5. Spread the nuts in the Air Fryer basket and spray them with cooking oil.
6. Air fry these nuts for 10 minutes and toss once cooked halfway through.
7. Serve.

Nutritional Values:

Calories: 295, Fat: 13.8g, Carb: 7g, Protein: 10g

TOASTED WALNUTS

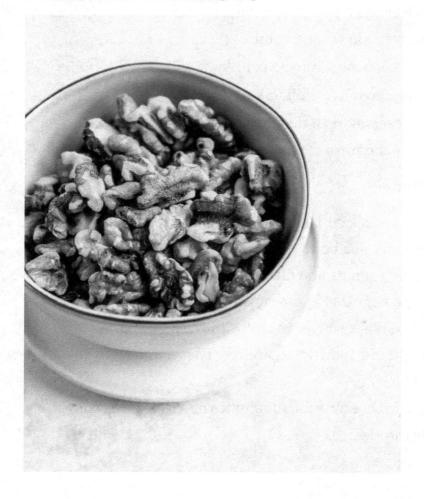

Serves: 6-8

Prep Time: 14 mins

Cook Time: 10 mins

Ingredients:

- 1/4 cup California walnuts

Directions:

1. At 350 degrees F, preheat your Air Fryer.
2. Grease the Air Fryer basket with vegetable oil.
3. Spread the walnuts in the Air Fryer basket and spray them with cooking oil.
4. Air fry these nuts for 10 minutes and toss once cooked halfway through.
5. Serve.

Nutritional Values:

Calories: 140, Fat: 16.3g, Carb: 5.7g, Protein: 18g

PEPPER ROASTED WALNUTS

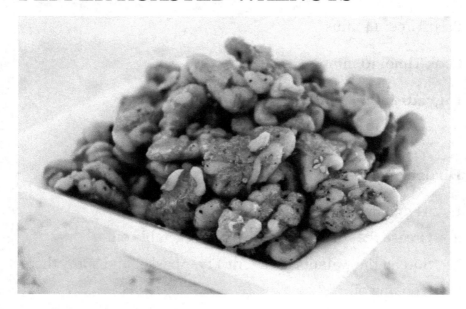

Prep Time: 14 mins

Cook Time: 10 mins

Ingredients:

- 1 cup shelled walnuts
- 1 tablespoon olive oil
- 1 teaspoon salt flakes
- 1/2 teaspoons black pepper

Directions:

1. Mix walnuts with oil, salt and black pepper in a bowl.
2. At 350 degrees F, preheat your Air Fryer.
3. Grease the Air Fryer basket with vegetable oil.
4. Spread the nuts in the Air Fryer basket and spray them with cooking oil.
5. Air fry these nuts for 10 minutes and toss once cooked halfway through.
6. Serve.

Nutritional Values:

Calories: 284, Fat: 16.3g, Carb: 8.3 g, Protein: 6g

CANDIED WALNUTS

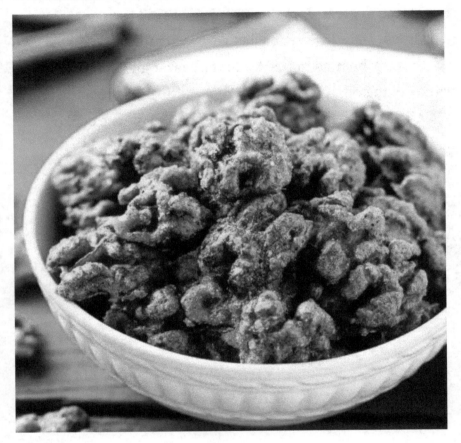

Serves: 6-8

Prep Time: 14 mins

Cook Time: 20 mins

Ingredients:

- 1/4 cup packed brown swerve
- 1 teaspoon Salt, to taste
- 1 teaspoon ground cinnamon
- 1/4 teaspoon ground cayenne
- 1 egg white
- 1 teaspoon vanilla extract
- 4 cups (12 oz.) raw walnut halves

Directions:

1. Mix swerve, salt, cinnamon, cayenne, egg white and vanilla in a bowl.
2. Toss in walnuts and mix well to coat.
3. At 300 degrees F, preheat your Air Fryer.
4. Grease the Air Fryer basket with vegetable oil.
5. Spread the nuts in the Air Fryer basket and spray them with cooking oil.
6. Air fry these nuts for 20 minutes and toss once cooked halfway through.
7. Serve.

Nutritional Values:

Calories: 144, Fat: 20g, Carb: 7g, Protein: 6g

ROASTED WALNUTS

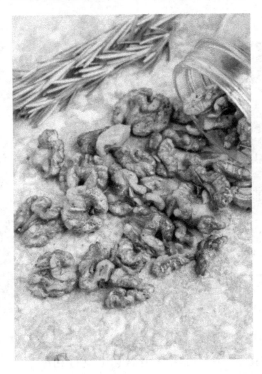

Serves: 6-8

Prep Time: 14 mins

Cook Time: 12 mins

Ingredients:

- 2 cups walnut pieces
- 1 tablespoon melted butter
- 1 teaspoon dried or fresh rosemary
- Salt to taste

Directions:

1. Mix walnuts with butter, rosemary and salt in a bowl.
2. At 375 degrees F, preheat your Air Fryer.
3. Grease the Air Fryer basket with vegetable oil.
4. Spread the nuts in the Air Fryer basket and spray them with cooking oil.
5. Air fry these nuts for 12 minutes and toss once cooked halfway through.
6. Serve.

Nutritional Values:

Calories: 157, Fat: 15g, Carb: 8.1g, Protein: 6g

CINNAMON ROASTED WALNUTS

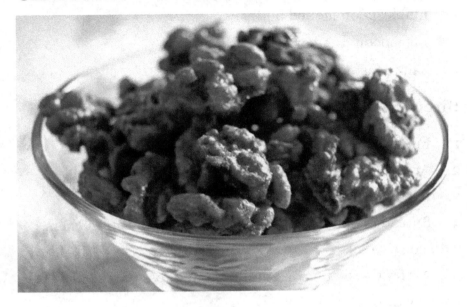

Serves: 6-8

Prep Time: 14 mins

Cook Time: 15 mins

Ingredients:

- 1 egg white
- 1 tablespoon water
- 1-pound walnut halves
- ¼ cup brown swerve

- 1½ teaspoons ground cinnamon
- 1 teaspoon salt
- ½ teaspoon allspice
- ½ teaspoon ground ginger

Directions:

1. Mix egg white, water, swerve, cinnamon, salt, allspice and ginger in a saucepan.
2. Cook this mixture to a boil and mix well.
3. Toss in pistachios and mix well to coat.
4. At 325 degrees F, preheat your Air Fryer.
5. Grease the Air Fryer basket with vegetable oil.
6. Spread the nuts in the Air Fryer basket and spray them with cooking oil.
7. Air fry these nuts for 15 minutes and toss once cooked halfway through.
8. Serve.

Nutritional Values:

Calories: 255, fat: 18g, carb: 3g, Protein: 20g

ROSEMARY TOASTED WALNUTS

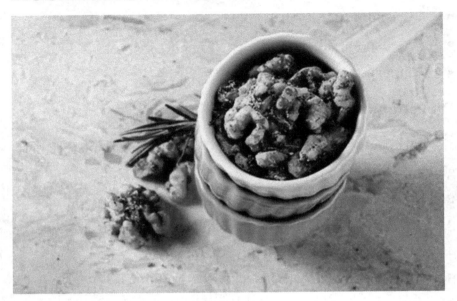

Serves: 6-8

Prep Time: 14 mins

Cook Time: 15 mins

Ingredients:

- 2 cups raw walnuts
- 2 tablespoons fresh rosemary, chopped
- 1/4 cup olive oil
- 1/2 teaspoon salt

- 1 teaspoon black pepper

Directions:

1. Mix rosemary with oil, black pepper and salt in a bowl.
2. At 350 degrees F, preheat your Air Fryer.
3. Grease the Air Fryer basket with vegetable oil.
4. Spread the nuts in the Air Fryer basket and spray them with cooking oil.
5. Air fry these nuts for 15 minutes and toss once cooked halfway through.
6. Serve.

Nutritional Values:

Calories: 134, Fat: 19.1g, Carb: 4.8g, Protein: 10g

MAPLE ROASTED WALNUTS

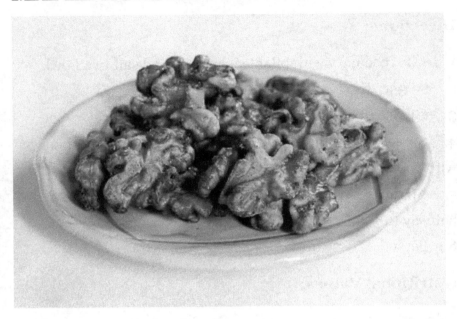

Serves: 6-8

Prep Time: 14 mins

Cook Time: 20 mins

Ingredients:

- 1 cup walnuts
- 2 tablespoon choc zero maple syrup
- ¼ cup swerve

- ½ teaspoons chili powder
- ½ teaspoons salt

Directions:

1. Mix maple syrup, swerve, chili powder and salt.
2. Toss in walnuts and mix well to coat.
3. At 350 degrees F, preheat your Air Fryer.
4. Grease the Air Fryer basket with vegetable oil.
5. Spread the nuts in the Air Fryer basket and spray them with cooking oil.
6. Air fry these nuts for 20 minutes and toss once cooked halfway through.
7. Serve.

Nutritional Values:

Calories: 395, Fat: 20.2g, Carb: 7g, Protein: 18g

ESPRESSO ROASTED WALNUTS

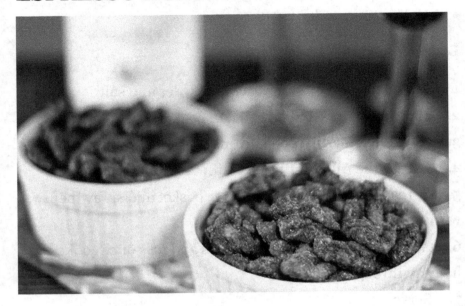

Serves: 6-8

Prep Time: 14 mins

Cook Time: 45 mins

Ingredients:

- 4 cups California walnuts
- 2 egg whites
- 1 teaspoon vanilla
- 3/4 cup brown swerve

- 2 tablespoons cocoa powder
- 2 teaspoons instant espresso powder
- 1 teaspoon of dried chipotle pepper
- 1/2 teaspoon salt

Directions:

1. Beat egg whites with vanilla, swerve, cocoa powder, espresso powder, chipotle pepper and salt in a bowl.
2. Toss in walnuts and mix well to coat.
3. At 275 degrees F, preheat your Air Fryer.
4. Grease the Air Fryer basket with vegetable oil.
5. Spread the nuts in the Air Fryer basket and spray them with cooking oil.
6. Air fry these nuts for 45 minutes and toss once cooked halfway through.
7. Serve.

Nutritional Values:

Calories: 132, Fat: 18g, Carb: 6.9g, Protein: 9g

ROSEMARY MACADAMIAS

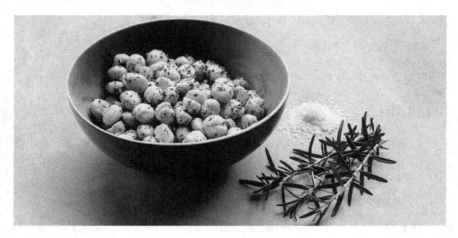

Serves: 6-8

Prep Time: 14 mins

Cook Time: 10 mins

Ingredients:

- 2 cups unsalted macadamias
- 1 tablespoon salt
- 3 tablespoons rosemary leaves, chopped
- 1 tablespoon macadamia oil

Directions:

1. Toss macadamias with oil, rosemary and salt in a bowl.

2. At 350 degrees F, preheat your Air Fryer.

3. Grease the Air Fryer basket with vegetable oil.

4. Spread the nuts in the Air Fryer basket and spray them with cooking oil.

5. Air fry these nuts for 10 minutes and toss once cooked halfway through.

6. Serve.

Nutritional Values:

Calories: 144, Fat: 16.3g, Carb: 5.9g, Protein: 6g

SPICED MACADAMIA NUTS

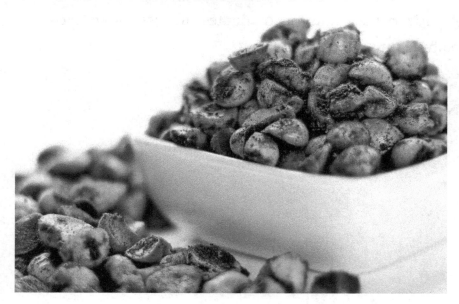

Serves: 6-8

Prep Time: 14 mins

Cook Time: 25 mins

Ingredients:

- 1 tablespoon vegetable oil

- 2 cups macadamia nuts
- 1 tablespoon swerve
- 1 teaspoon curry powder
- 1 teaspoon ground cumin
- 1 teaspoon ground coriander
- 1 teaspoon chili powder
- 1 teaspoon salt
- 1/2 teaspoons cayenne pepper

Directions:

1. Mix cayenne pepper, salt, chili powder, cumin, curry powder, swerve and oil in a bowl.
2. Toss in macadamia nuts and mix well to coat.
3. At 250 degrees F, preheat your Air Fryer.
4. Grease the Air Fryer basket with vegetable oil.
5. Spread the nuts in the Air Fryer basket and spray them with cooking oil.
6. Air fry these nuts for 25 minutes and toss once cooked halfway through.
7. Serve.

Nutritional Values:

Calories: 140, Fat: 16g, Carb: 6.2g, Protein: 6g

CHILE MACADAMIA NUTS

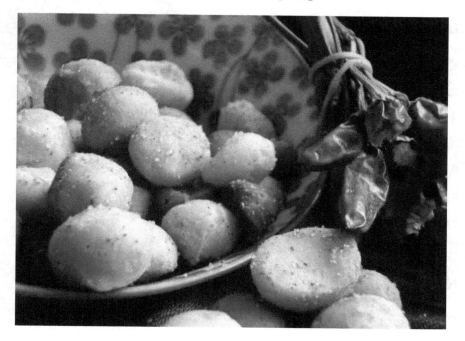

Serves: 6-8

Prep Time: 14 mins

Cook Time: 25 mins

Ingredients:

- 2 cups raw shelled macadamia nuts
- 1 teaspoon canola oil
- 1 1/2 teaspoons chili powder

- 1 teaspoon salt

Directions:

1. Mix chili powder, salt, oil and macadamia nuts in a bowl.
2. At 300 degrees F, preheat your Air Fryer.
3. Grease the Air Fryer basket with vegetable oil.
4. Spread the nuts in the Air Fryer basket and spray them with cooking oil.
5. Air fry these nuts for 25 minutes and toss once cooked halfway through.
6. Serve.

Nutritional Values:

Calories: 295, Fat: 14.9g, Carb: 4.8g, Protein: 18g

MAPLE MACADAMIA NUTS

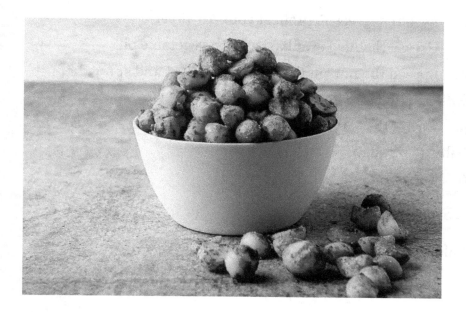

Serves: 6-8

Prep Time: 14 mins

Cook Time: 8 mins

Ingredients:

- 1 cup of macadamia nuts
- 1/4 cup choc zero maple syrup
- Pinch of salt

Directions:

1. Mix macadamia nuts with maple syrup and salt in a bowl.
2. At 350 degrees F, preheat your Air Fryer.
3. Grease the Air Fryer basket with vegetable oil.
4. Spread the nuts in the Air Fryer basket and spray them with cooking oil.
5. Air fry these nuts for 8 minutes and toss once cooked halfway through.
6. Serve.

Nutritional Values:

Calories: 288, Fat: 17.1g, Carb: 7.9g, Protein: 10g

ROSEMARY BRAZIL NUTS

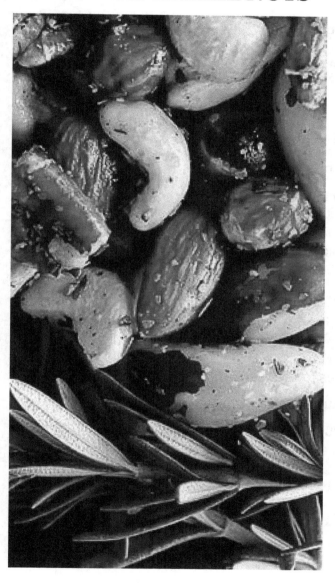

Serves: 6-8

Prep Time: 14 mins

Cook Time: 17 mins

Ingredients:

- 2 cups raw brazil nuts
- 1 tablespoon olive oil
- 1/4 cup fresh rosemary, chopped
- ½ teaspoons salt
- ½ teaspoons cayenne pepper

Directions:

1. Mix brazil nuts with oil, rosemary, cayenne pepper and salt in a bowl.
2. At 375 degrees F, preheat your Air Fryer.
3. Grease the Air Fryer basket with vegetable oil.
4. Spread the nuts in the Air Fryer basket and spray them with cooking oil.
5. Air fry these nuts for 17 minutes and toss once cooked halfway through.
6. Serve.

Nutritional Values:

Calories: 134, Fat: 20g, Carb: 7g, Protein: 6g

BRAZIL NUTS MIX

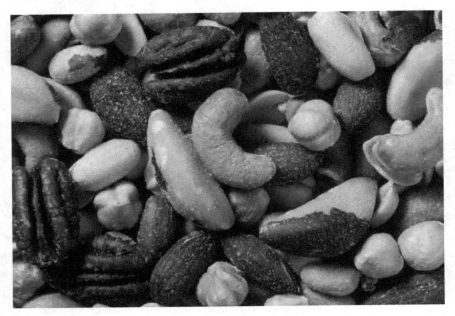

Serves: 6-8

Prep Time: 14 mins

Cook Time: 25 mins

Ingredients:

- 1 cup pecans
- 1 cup walnuts
- 2 cups brazil nuts

- 1/2 cup raw almonds
- 1 tablespoon fresh rosemary leaves
- 1 tablespoon fresh thyme leaves
- 1/2 tablespoons parsley chopped
- 1 teaspoon garlic granules
- 1/2 teaspoon paprika
- 1/2 teaspoon salt
- 1/4 teaspoon ground black pepper
- 1/2 tablespoons olive oil

Directions:

1. Mix rosemary, parsley, thyme, garlic, paprika, salt, black pepper and oil in a bowl.
2. Toss in nuts and mix well to coat.
3. At 350 degrees F, preheat your Air Fryer.
4. Grease the Air Fryer basket with vegetable oil.
5. Spread the nuts in the Air Fryer basket and spray them with cooking oil.
6. Air fry these nuts for 25 minutes and toss once cooked halfway through.
7. Serve.

Nutritional Values:

Calories: 157, Fat: 16.3g, Carb: 4.8g, Protein: 9g

ESPRESSO ROASTED CASHEWS

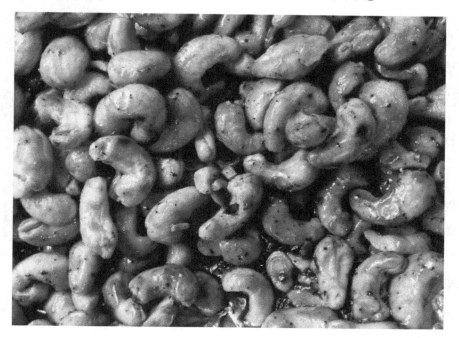

Serves: 6-8

Prep Time: 14 mins

Cook Time: 45 mins

Ingredients:

- 4 cups California cashews
- 2 egg whites
- 1 teaspoon vanilla

- 3/4 cup brown swerve
- 2 tablespoons cocoa powder
- 2 teaspoons instant espresso powder
- 1 teaspoon of dried chipotle pepper
- 1/2 teaspoon salt

Directions:

1. Beat egg whites with vanilla, swerve, cocoa powder, espresso powder, chipotle pepper and salt in a bowl.
2. Toss in cashews and mix well to coat.
3. At 275 degrees F, preheat your Air Fryer.
4. Grease the Air Fryer basket with vegetable oil.
5. Spread the nuts in the Air Fryer basket and spray them with cooking oil.
6. Air fry these nuts for 45 minutes and toss once cooked halfway through.
7. Serve.

Nutritional Values:

Calories: 144, Fat: 18g, Carb: 8.3 g, Protein: 6g

CHILE BRAZILIAN NUTS

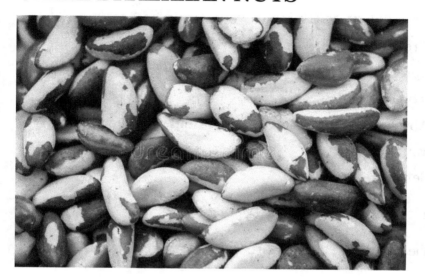

Serves: 6-8

Prep Time: 14 mins

Cook Time: 25 mins

Ingredients:

- 2 cups raw Brazilian nuts
- 1 teaspoon canola oil
- 1 1⁄2 teaspoons chili powder
- 1 teaspoon salt

Directions:

1. Mix chili powder, salt, oil and Brazilian nuts in a bowl.
2. At 300 degrees F, preheat your Air Fryer.
3. Grease the Air Fryer basket with vegetable oil.
4. Spread the nuts in the Air Fryer basket and spray them with cooking oil.
5. Air fry these nuts for 25 minutes and toss once cooked halfway through.
6. Serve.

Nutritional Values:

Calories: 131, Fat: 20.2g, Carb: 5.9g, Protein: 18g

GARLIC MACADAMIA NUTS

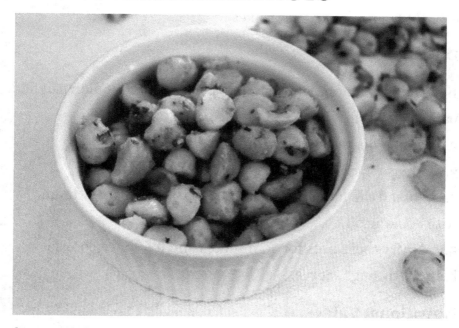

Serves: 6-8

Prep Time: 14 mins

Cook Time: 10 mins

Ingredients:

- 1 cup roasted macadamia nuts
- 1/2 teaspoons olive oil
- 1/2 teaspoons garlic powder

- 1/2 teaspoons onion salt
- 1/4 teaspoons parsley flakes

Directions:

1. Mix macadamia nuts with oil, garlic powder, onion salt and parsley flakes in a bowl.
2. At 350 degrees F, preheat your Air Fryer.
3. Grease the Air Fryer basket with vegetable oil.
4. Spread the nuts in the Air Fryer basket and spray them with cooking oil.
5. Air fry these nuts for 10 minutes and toss once cooked halfway through. Serve.

Nutritional Values:

Calories: 157, Fat: 16.3g, Carb: 5.7g, Protein: 6g

CHAI SPICED NUTS

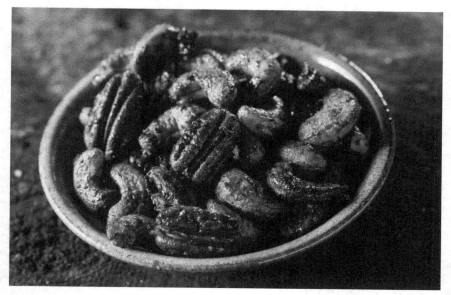

Serves: 6-8

Prep Time: 14 mins

Cook Time: 30 mins

Ingredients:

- For the chai spice
- 1 teaspoon ground cinnamon
- ½ teaspoons ground ginger
- ¼ teaspoons ground nutmeg

- ¼ teaspoons ground allspice
- ⅛ teaspoons ground cloves
- 1 large pinch salt
- Seeds from 6 cardamom pods
- For the nuts
- 1 egg white
- ½ teaspoons vanilla extract
- ½ cup soft swerve (light)
- ½ cup almonds
- ½ cup pecan nuts
- ⅜ cup cashew nuts
- ⅜ cup hazelnuts

Directions:

1. Beat egg white with swerve and vanilla in a bowl.
2. Toss in nuts and mix well to coat.
3. At 350 degrees F, preheat your Air Fryer.
4. Grease the Air Fryer basket with vegetable oil.
5. Spread the nuts in the Air Fryer basket and spray them with cooking oil.
6. Air fry these nuts for 30 minutes and toss once cooked halfway through.

7. Mix all the chai spice ingredients in a bowl.

8. Toss in candied nuts and mix well.

9. Serve.

Nutritional Values:

Calories: 288, Fat: 13.8g, Carb: 7.7g, Protein: 10g

GINGERBREAD GLAZED NUTS

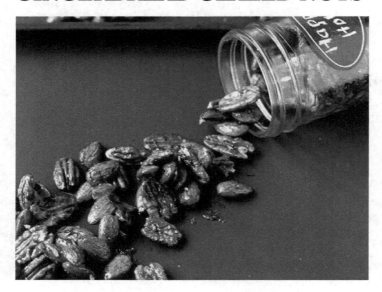

Serves: 6-8

Prep Time: 14 mins

Cook Time: 10 mins

Ingredients:

- 1½ cups almonds
- 1½ cup pecans
- 1 teaspoon coconut oil
- 2 tablespoons choc zero maple syrup

- ½ teaspoons ground cinnamon
- 2 teaspoons ginger

Directions:

1. Mix pecans, almonds, oil, maple syrup, cinnamon and ginger in a bowl.
2. At 350 degrees F, preheat your Air Fryer.
3. Grease the Air Fryer basket with vegetable oil.
4. Spread the nuts in the Air Fryer basket and spray them with cooking oil.
5. Air fry these nuts for 10 minutes and toss once cooked halfway through.
6. Serve.

Nutritional Values:

Calories: 134, Fat: 16.3g, Carb: 6.2g, Protein: 9g

SESAME CASHEW CLUSTERS

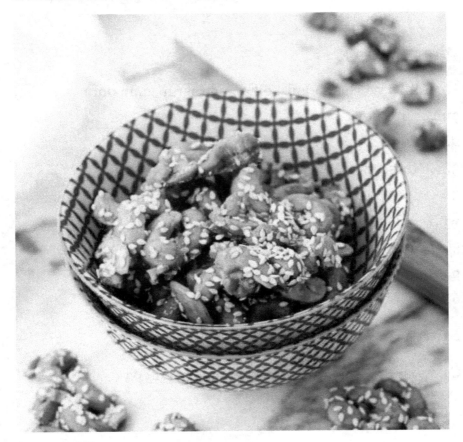

Serves: 6-8

Prep Time: 14 mins

Cook Time: 10 mins

Ingredients:

- 1 cup whole cashews
- 2 tablespoons choc zero maple syrup
- 1/4 teaspoons 1/8 teaspoons salt
- 1 tablespoon toasted sesame seeds

Directions:

1. Mix cashews with maple syrup, and salt in a bowl.
2. At 300 degrees F, preheat your Air Fryer.
3. Grease the Air Fryer basket with vegetable oil.
4. Spread the nuts in the Air Fryer basket and drizzle sesame seeds on top.
5. Air fry these nuts for 10 minutes and toss once cooked halfway through.
6. Serve.

Nutritional Values:

Calories: 144, Fat: 19.1g, Carb: 8.1g, Protein: 6g

CHILLI LIME CASHEWS

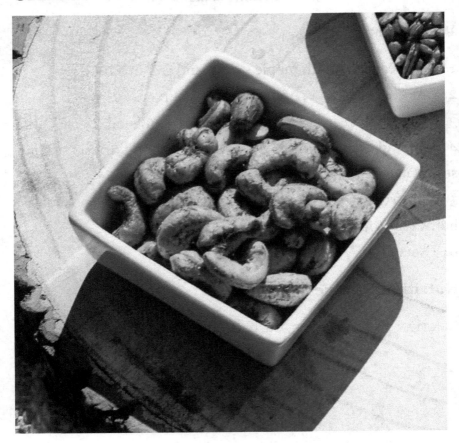

Serves: 6-8

Prep Time: 14 mins

Cook Time: 25 mins

Ingredients:

- 2-1/2 cups cashews, roasted, salted
- 1/4 cup olive oil
- 1 tablespoon chili powder
- 1/2 teaspoon cayenne pepper
- Zest from 1 lime
- 2 tablespoons lime juice

Directions:

1. Mix cashews with oil, chili powder, cayenne pepper, lime zest and juice in a bowl.
2. At 350 degrees F, preheat your Air Fryer.
3. Grease the Air Fryer basket with vegetable oil.
4. Spread the nuts in the Air Fryer basket and spray them with cooking oil.
5. Air fry these nuts for 25 minutes and toss once cooked halfway through.
6. Serve.

Nutritional Values:

Calories: 283, Fat: 20g, Carb: 7g, Protein: 18g

CHOCOLATE PECANS

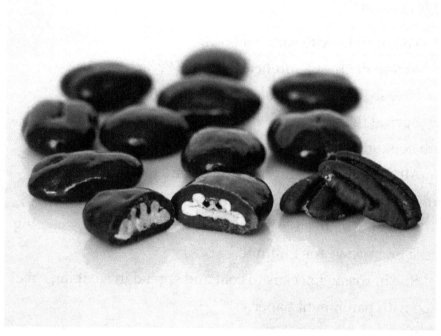

Serves: 6-8

Prep Time: 14 mins

Cook Time: 11 mins

Ingredients:

- 2 cups pecans
- 1 cup dark chocolate chips
- 1 teaspoon coconut oil
- Kosher or salt

Directions:

1. Toss pecans with salt in a bowl.
2. At 350 degrees F, preheat your Air Fryer.
3. Grease the Air Fryer basket with vegetable oil.
4. Spread the nuts in the Air Fryer basket and spray them with cooking oil.
5. Air fry these nuts for 10 minutes and toss once cooked halfway through.
6. Melt chocolate chips, and coconut oil in a bowl by heating in the microwave for 1 minute.
7. Stir in roasted pecans to coat and spread in a baking sheet lined with parchment paper.
8. Serve.

Nutritional Values:

Calories: 132, Fat: 10g, Carb: 8g, Protein: 6g

CHOCOLATE DIPPED WALNUTS

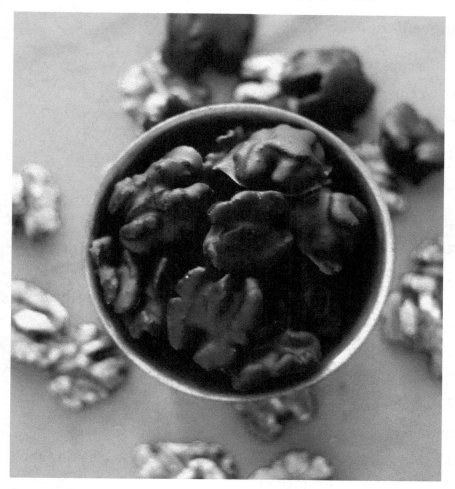

Serves: 6-8

Prep Time: 14 mins

Cook Time: 11 mins

Ingredients:

- 2 cups walnuts
- 1 cup chocolate chips dark
- 1 teaspoon coconut oil
- Kosher or salt

Directions:

1. Toss walnuts with salt in a bowl.
2. At 350 degrees F, preheat your Air Fryer.
3. Grease the Air Fryer basket with vegetable oil.
4. Spread the nuts in the Air Fryer basket and spray them with cooking oil.
5. Air fry these nuts for 10 minutes and toss once cooked halfway through.
6. Melt chocolate chips, and coconut oil in a bowl by heating in the microwave for 1 minute.
7. Stir in roasted walnuts to coat and spread in a baking sheet lined with parchment paper.
8. Serve.

Nutritional Values:

Calories: 157, Fat: 17.1g, Carb: 7g, Protein: 6g

CHOCOLATE DIPPED CASHEWS

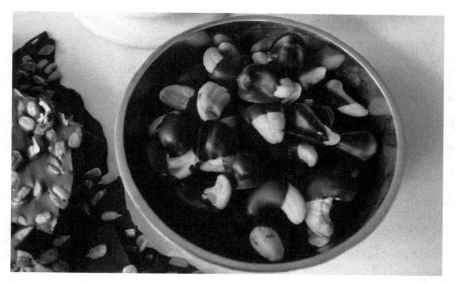

Serves: 6-8

Prep Time: 14 mins

Cook Time: 11 mins

Ingredients:

- 2 cups cashews
- 1 cup dark chocolate chips

- 1 teaspoon coconut oil
- Kosher or salt

Directions:

1. Toss cashews with salt in a bowl.

2. At 350 degrees F, preheat your Air Fryer.

3. Grease the Air Fryer basket with vegetable oil.

4. Spread the nuts in the Air Fryer basket and spray them with cooking oil.

5. Air fry these nuts for 10 minutes and toss once cooked halfway through.

6. Melt chocolate chips, and coconut oil in a bowl by heating in the microwave for 1 minute.

7. Stir in roasted cashews to coat and spread in a baking sheet lined with parchment paper.

8. Serve.

Nutritional Values:

Calories: 121, Fat: 16.3g, Carb: 6.9g, Protein: 10g

CHOCOLATE BRAZIL NUTS

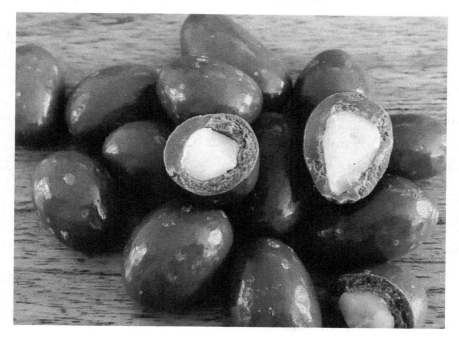

Serves: 6-8

Prep Time: 14 mins

Cook Time: 11 mins

Ingredients:

- 2 cups brazil nuts
- 1 cup dark chocolate chips
- 1 teaspoon coconut oil

- Kosher or salt

Directions:

1. Toss brazil nuts with salt in a bowl.
2. At 350 degrees F, preheat your Air Fryer.
3. Grease the Air Fryer basket with vegetable oil.
4. Spread the nuts in the Air Fryer basket and spray them with cooking oil.
5. Air fry these nuts for 10 minutes and toss once cooked halfway through.
6. Melt chocolate chips, and coconut oil in a bowl by heating in the microwave for 1 minute.
7. Stir in roasted brazil nuts to coat and spread in a baking sheet lined with parchment paper.
8. Serve.

Nutritional Values:

Calories: 134, Fat: 17.4g, Carb: 8.3 g, Protein: 9g

CHOCOLATE PISTACHIOS

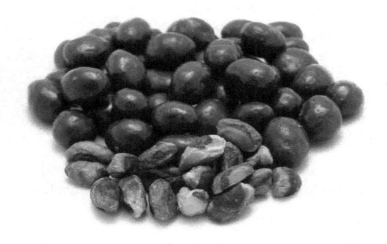

Serves: 6-8

Prep Time: 14 mins

Cook Time: 11 mins

Ingredients:

- 2 cups pistachios, shelled
- 1 cup dark chocolate chips
- 1 teaspoon coconut oil

- Kosher or salt

Directions:

1. Toss pistachios with salt in a bowl.
2. At 350 degrees F, preheat your Air Fryer.
3. Grease the Air Fryer basket with vegetable oil.
4. Spread the nuts in the Air Fryer basket and spray them with cooking oil.
5. Air fry these nuts for 10 minutes and toss once cooked halfway through.
6. Melt chocolate chips, and coconut oil in a bowl by heating in the microwave for 1 minute.
7. Stir in roasted pistachios to coat and spread in a baking sheet lined with parchment paper.
8. Serve.

Nutritional Values:

Calories: 195, Fat: 18g, Carb: 4.8g, Protein: 18g

CHOCOLATE MACADAMIA NUTS

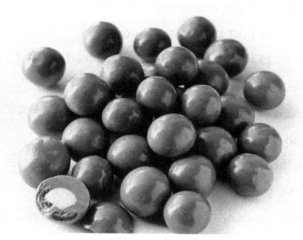

Serves: 6-8

Prep Time: 14 mins

Cook Time: 11 mins

Ingredients:

- 2 cups macadamia nuts
- 1 cup dark chocolate chips

- 1 teaspoon coconut oil
- Kosher or salt

Directions:

1. Toss macadamia nuts with salt in a bowl.
2. At 350 degrees F, preheat your Air Fryer.
3. Grease the Air Fryer basket with vegetable oil.
4. Spread the nuts in the Air Fryer basket and spray them with cooking oil.
5. Air fry these nuts for 10 minutes and toss once cooked halfway through.
6. Melt chocolate chips, and coconut oil in a bowl by heating in the microwave for 1 minute.
7. Stir in roasted macadamia nuts to coat and spread in a baking sheet lined with parchment paper.
8. Serve.

Nutritional Values:

Calories: 288, Fat: 10g, Carb: 6.2g, Protein: 6g

CHOCOLATE DIPPED PEANUTS

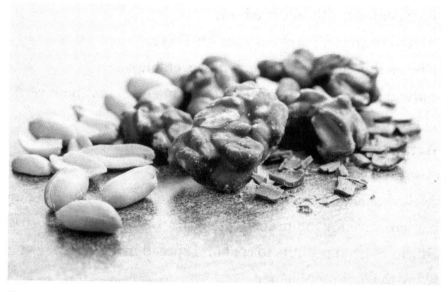

Serves: 6-8

Prep Time: 14 mins

Cook Time: 14 mins

Ingredients:

- 2 cups peanuts, peeled
- 1 cup dark chocolate chips
- 1 teaspoon coconut oil
- Kosher or salt

Directions:

1. Toss peanuts with salt in a bowl.
2. At 350 degrees F, preheat your Air Fryer.
3. Grease the Air Fryer basket with vegetable oil.
4. Spread the nuts in the Air Fryer basket and spray them with cooking oil.
5. Air fry these nuts for 10 minutes and toss once cooked halfway through.
6. Melt chocolate chips, and coconut oil in a bowl by heating in the microwave for 1 minute.
7. Stir in roasted peanuts to coat and spread in a baking sheet lined with parchment paper.
8. Serve.

Nutritional Values:

Calories: 144, Fat: 20.2g, Carb: 8.1g, Protein: 6g

CPSIA information can be obtained
at www.ICGtesting.com
Printed in the USA
BVHW091921230621
610293BV00007B/868